THE ULTIMATE FATTY LIVER RECIPE COOKBOOK

Delicious, Healthy Meals to Support Your Liver Health

Ellis Kay

INTRODUCTION

Explanation of Fatty Liver Disease and Its Causes

Fatty liver disease, also known as hepatic steatosis, is a condition where fat accumulates in the liver. This can occur in people who consume excessive amounts of alcohol, known as alcoholic fatty liver disease, or in those who do not drink alcohol excessively, known as non-alcoholic fatty liver disease (NAFLD).

NAFLD is becoming increasingly common, affecting approximately 25% of the global population. The exact cause of NAFLD is not known, but several risk factors have been identified. These include obesity, insulin resistance, metabolic syndrome, type 2 diabetes, and high levels of triglycerides in the blood.

When fat accumulates in the liver, it can cause inflammation and damage to liver cells, leading to fibrosis (scarring) and cirrhosis. Cirrhosis is a severe liver disease that can lead to liver failure and the need for a liver transplant.

The diagnosis of fatty liver disease is made through blood tests, imaging studies such as ultrasound or CT scans, and liver biopsy. Treatment involves lifestyle changes such as losing weight, exercising regularly, avoiding alcohol and certain medications, and following a healthy diet. In severe cases, medication or surgery may be required.

Importance of a Healthy Diet in Managing Fatty Liver Disease

A healthy diet is essential in managing fatty liver disease, particularly for those with NAFLD. The goal of a healthy diet is to reduce inflammation in the liver, improve insulin sensitivity, and promote weight loss.

A healthy diet for fatty liver disease should include whole, unprocessed foods such as fruits, vegetables, whole grains, lean proteins, and healthy fats. Foods to avoid include high-sugar and high-fat foods, processed foods, and alcohol.

There are several specific dietary recommendations for managing fatty liver disease, including:

1. **Reducing calorie intake:** Losing weight is one of the most effective ways to improve liver function in people with fatty liver disease. Reducing calorie intake by 500-1000 calories per day can lead to significant weight loss and improve liver function.

2. **Increasing fiber intake:** Fiber-rich foods such as fruits, vegetables, and whole grains can help improve insulin sensitivity and reduce inflammation in the liver.

3. **Limiting saturated and trans fats:** Foods high in saturated and trans fats, such as fried foods, fatty meats, and processed snacks, can increase inflammation in the liver.

4. **Limiting sugar and refined carbohydrates:** Foods high in sugar and refined carbohydrates, such as candy, soda, and white bread, can increase insulin resistance and contribute to inflammation in the

liver.

5. **Avoiding alcohol:** Alcohol can worsen liver inflammation and damage in people with fatty liver disease.

Following a healthy diet can not only improve liver function but also lead to other health benefits such as improved cardiovascular health and weight loss.

Overview of the Cookbook and Its Purpose

The cookbook is a collection of recipes specifically designed for people with fatty liver disease. The purpose of the cookbook is to provide healthy and delicious meal options that can help manage fatty liver disease.

The cookbook includes a variety of recipes for breakfast, lunch, dinner, and snacks, all of which are low in saturated and trans fats, high in fiber, and low in sugar and refined carbohydrates. The recipes feature whole, unprocessed foods such as fruits, vegetables, whole grains, and lean proteins.

In addition to recipes, the cookbook includes information on the importance of a healthy diet in managing fatty liver disease, as well as tips for meal planning and grocery shopping. The cookbook is designed to be user-friendly and accessible to people with all levels of cooking experience.

By following the recipes in the cookbook and making healthy dietary changes, people with fatty liver disease can improve liver function, reduce inflammation, and promote overall health and well-being. The cookbook can also be a helpful resource for people looking to prevent fatty liver disease or improve their overall health.

The recipes in the cookbook are not only healthy but also

delicious and easy to make. Some examples of recipes in the cookbook include roasted vegetable quinoa bowls, grilled chicken and vegetable skewers, and berry and yogurt parfaits. Each recipe includes detailed instructions and nutritional information, making it easy for people to make informed decisions about their diet.

CHAPTER ONE

*Understanding Fatty
Liver Disease*

Explanation Of Fatty Liver Disease And Its Types

Fatty liver disease is a condition in which there is an accumulation of excess fat in the liver cells. This condition is also known as hepatic steatosis. The liver is an important organ in the body that performs a wide range of functions, including the metabolism of fats, proteins, and carbohydrates, as well as the production of bile, which aids in the digestion of fats. When there is too much fat in the liver, it can interfere with its ability to function properly.

There are two types of fatty liver disease: alcoholic fatty liver disease and nonalcoholic fatty liver disease (NAFLD). Alcoholic fatty liver disease is caused by excessive alcohol consumption, while NAFLD is not related to alcohol consumption. NAFLD is more common and can be caused by factors such as obesity, insulin resistance, high blood pressure, high levels of triglycerides, and metabolic syndrome.

NAFLD can also be further divided into two types: nonalcoholic fatty liver (NAFL) and nonalcoholic steatohepatitis (NASH). NAFL is characterized by the accumulation of excess fat in the liver cells, but it does not cause inflammation or liver damage. NASH, on the other hand, is a more severe form of NAFLD in which there is inflammation and liver damage in addition to the accumulation of excess fat in the liver cells. NASH can lead to cirrhosis, liver failure, and liver cancer if left untreated.

Symptoms Of Fatty Liver Disease

In the early stages, fatty liver disease may not cause any noticeable symptoms. However, as the condition progresses, some common symptoms may include:

- Fatigue
- Weakness
- Abdominal pain
- Loss of appetite
- Nausea and vomiting
- Jaundice (yellowing of the skin and eyes)
- Swelling in the legs and ankles
- Mental confusion

It is important to note that not everyone with fatty liver disease will experience symptoms. Some people may only find out they have the condition after a routine blood test or imaging study.

Risk Factors And Causes Of Fatty Liver Disease

There are several risk factors that can increase the likelihood of developing fatty liver disease. These include:

- Obesity: Excess body weight, especially in the abdomen, can increase the risk of NAFLD.

- Insulin resistance: This occurs when the body is unable to use insulin properly, which can lead to high blood sugar levels and an increased risk of NAFLD.

- High levels of triglycerides: Triglycerides are a type of fat found in the blood. High levels can increase the risk of NAFLD.

- Metabolic syndrome: This is a cluster of conditions that includes obesity, high blood pressure, high blood sugar levels, and high levels of triglycerides. Having metabolic syndrome can increase the risk of NAFLD.

- Type 2 diabetes: This condition is characterized by high blood sugar levels and insulin resistance, which can increase the risk of NAFLD.

- Excessive alcohol consumption: This can cause alcoholic fatty liver disease.

- Certain medications: Some medications, such as corticosteroids and tamoxifen, can increase the risk of NAFLD.

The Importance Of Dietary Changes In Managing Fatty Liver Disease

Making dietary changes can be an important part of managing fatty liver disease. The goal of dietary changes is to reduce the amount of fat in the liver and improve liver function. Here are some dietary changes that may be recommended:

- Weight loss: Losing weight can help reduce the amount of fat in the liver. A healthy weight loss goal is 1-2 pounds per week. It is important to achieve weight loss through a combination of diet and exercise.

- Reduced calorie intake: Consuming fewer calories can help with weight loss and reduce the amount of fat in the liver. This can be achieved by eating smaller portions, choosing lower-calorie foods, and limiting high-calorie foods and beverages such as sugary drinks and snacks.

- Limiting saturated and trans fats: These types of fats can contribute to the accumulation of fat in the liver. To reduce intake, choose lean protein sources such as fish, poultry, and legumes, and limit or avoid high-fat foods such as red meat, cheese, and butter.

- Increasing fiber intake: Fiber can help improve liver function and reduce inflammation. Good sources of fiber include fruits, vegetables, whole grains, and legumes.

- Limiting or avoiding alcohol: Excessive alcohol consumption can contribute to the development of fatty liver disease. It is important to limit alcohol intake or avoid it altogether to prevent further liver damage.

- Consulting with a registered dietitian: A registered dietitian can provide personalized recommendations and guidance on dietary changes to manage fatty liver disease.

It is important to note that dietary changes alone may not be sufficient to manage fatty liver disease. Other lifestyle changes, such as regular exercise and quitting smoking, as well as medical treatments, may also be necessary to improve liver function and prevent complications. It is important to work closely with a healthcare provider to develop an individualized treatment plan.

CHAPTER TWO

Overview Of A Healthy Diet For Fatty Liver Disease

Fatty liver disease is a condition in which fat builds up in the liver. This can lead to inflammation and damage to the liver. A healthy diet is essential for managing fatty liver disease. A healthy diet can help reduce inflammation, improve liver function, and prevent further damage to the liver.

A healthy diet for fatty liver disease should be low in saturated and trans fats and high in fruits, vegetables, whole grains, and lean proteins. It should also be low in sugar and refined carbohydrates. A healthy diet should be accompanied by regular exercise and weight management.

Foods to Include in the Diet

There are several foods that are beneficial for people with fatty liver disease. These include:

- **Fruits and Vegetables**: Fruits and vegetables are high in fiber, vitamins, and minerals. They are also low in calories and fat. Fruits and vegetables can help reduce inflammation, improve liver function, and prevent further damage to the liver. Aim for at least five servings of fruits and vegetables per day.

- **Whole Grains**: Whole grains are high in fiber and complex carbohydrates. They can help regulate blood sugar and insulin levels, which is important for people with fatty liver disease. Whole grains can also help reduce inflammation and improve liver function. Examples of whole grains include brown rice, quinoa, whole wheat bread, and oatmeal.

- **Lean Proteins**: Lean proteins are important for building and repairing tissues in the body. They are also low in saturated fat, which is important for people with fatty liver disease. Examples of lean proteins include chicken, turkey, fish, beans, and tofu.

- **Healthy Fats**: Healthy fats, such as those found in nuts, seeds, and avocado, can help reduce inflammation and improve liver function. These fats are also important for overall health and well-being.

Foods to Avoid in the Diet

There are several foods that should be avoided or limited in a healthy diet for fatty liver disease. These include:

- **Saturated and Trans Fats**: Saturated and trans fats can contribute to inflammation and damage to the liver. These fats are found in foods such as red meat, butter, cheese, and fried foods.

- **Sugar and Refined Carbohydrates**: Sugar and refined carbohydrates can contribute to insulin resistance, which is a risk factor for fatty liver disease. These foods are found in sugary drinks, candy, pastries, and white bread.

- **Alcohol**: Alcohol can cause inflammation and

damage to the liver. It is important to avoid or limit alcohol consumption for people with fatty liver disease.

Importance Of Portion Control And Meal Timing

Portion control and meal timing are important aspects of a healthy diet for fatty liver disease. Eating large meals or snacking throughout the day can contribute to weight gain and insulin resistance, which are risk factors for fatty liver disease. It is important to eat regular meals and snacks that are balanced and nutrient-dense.

Portion control is also important for managing weight and reducing inflammation. It is recommended to use smaller plates and bowls to help with portion control. Eating slowly and paying attention to hunger and fullness cues can also help with portion control.

Meal timing can also have an impact on liver function. Eating regular meals and snacks can help regulate blood sugar and insulin levels. It is recommended to eat breakfast within an hour of waking up and to eat dinner at least two to three hours before bedtime.

CHAPTER THREE

Recipes for Breakfast

Introduction to breakfast recipes for fatty liver disease

Grilled Salmon with Poached Eggs and Avocado

This meal is a delicious combination of healthy fats, protein, and fiber. The grilled salmon provides omega-3 fatty acids, while the poached eggs add protein and the avocado provides healthy fats.

Ingredients:

- 2 salmon fillets
- 4 eggs
- 1 avocado
- Salt and pepper to taste

Instructions:

1. Preheat your grill to medium heat.
2. Season the salmon fillets with salt and pepper and place them on the grill. Cook for 10-12 minutes, flipping once.
3. While the salmon is cooking, poach the eggs in a pot of simmering water.
4. Cut the avocado in half, remove the pit, and slice it thinly.

5. Once the salmon is cooked, remove it from the grill and place it on a plate.

6. Place the poached eggs on top of the salmon and arrange the avocado slices on the side.

7. Serve and enjoy!

Nutritional Information:

This meal contains approximately 500 calories, 40 grams of protein, and 30 grams of healthy fats.

Quinoa Breakfast Bowl with Spinach, Mushrooms, and Tomato

This meal is a delicious and healthy breakfast option that is packed with protein and fiber. The quinoa provides a great source of protein, while the spinach, mushrooms, and tomato provide fiber and essential vitamins.

Ingredients:

- 1 cup quinoa
- 2 cups water
- 1 cup spinach
- 1 cup sliced mushrooms
- 1 cup cherry tomatoes, halved
- 1 tablespoon olive oil
- Salt and pepper to taste

Instructions:

1. Rinse the quinoa under cold water and place it in a pot with 2 cups of water. Bring to a boil, then reduce the heat to low and let simmer for 15-20 minutes, or until the water has been absorbed.

2. In a separate pan, heat the olive oil over medium heat. Add the mushrooms and cook until they are tender and browned, about 5-7 minutes.

3. Add the spinach to the pan and cook until it is wilted, about 1-2 minutes.

4. Once the quinoa is cooked, divide it evenly between two bowls.

5. Top the quinoa with the sautéed mushrooms and spinach, and the cherry tomatoes.

6. Season with salt and pepper to taste.

7. Serve and enjoy!

Nutritional Information:

This meal contains approximately 400 calories, 16 grams of protein, and 18 grams of healthy fats.

Oatmeal with Mixed Berries and Flaxseed

This meal is a classic and healthy breakfast option that is rich in fiber and antioxidants. The oatmeal provides a great source of fiber, while the mixed berries add antioxidants and the flaxseed provides omega-3 fatty acids.

Ingredients:

- 1 cup rolled oats
- 2 cups water
- 1 cup mixed berries (strawberries, blueberries, raspberries)
- 1 tablespoon flaxseed
- 1 tablespoon honey

Instructions:

1. In a pot, bring the water to a boil. Add the oats and reduce the heat to low. Cook for 5-7 minutes, stirring occasionally, until the oatmeal is thick and creamy.

2. Add the mixed berries to the pot and stir until they are heated through.

3. Divide the oatmeal evenly between two bowls.

4. Top the oatmeal with the flaxseed and drizzle with honey.

5. Serve and enjoy!

Nutritional Information:

This meal contains approximately 300 calories, 8 grams of protein.

Greek Yogurt with Chopped Nuts and Fruit

This meal is a healthy and filling breakfast option that is rich in protein and essential vitamins. The Greek yogurt provides a great source of protein, while the chopped nuts add healthy fats and the fruit provides essential vitamins and minerals.

Ingredients:

- 1 cup plain Greek yogurt
- 1/4 cup chopped nuts (almonds, walnuts, pecans)
- 1 cup chopped fruit (strawberries, blueberries, banana)
- 1 tablespoon honey

Instructions:

1. In a bowl, spoon the Greek yogurt.

2. Add the chopped nuts and fruit on top of the yogurt.

3. Drizzle with honey.

4. Serve and enjoy!

Nutritional Information:

This meal contains approximately 300 calories, 20 grams of protein, and 15 grams of healthy fats.

Vegetable Frittata with Sweet Potato Hash

This meal is a hearty and healthy breakfast option that is packed with protein and fiber. The frittata provides a great source of protein, while the sweet potato hash adds fiber and essential vitamins.

Ingredients:

- 6 eggs
- 1/2 cup milk
- 1/2 cup chopped vegetables (bell pepper, onion, zucchini)
- Salt and pepper to taste
- 1 tablespoon olive oil
- 1 sweet potato, peeled and diced
- 1/2 teaspoon paprika

Instructions:

1. Preheat your oven to 350°F.

2. In a bowl, whisk together the eggs, milk, chopped vegetables, salt, and pepper.

3. In a cast-iron skillet, heat the olive oil over medium heat. Add the sweet potato and cook until

it is tender and browned, about 10-12 minutes.

4. Sprinkle the paprika over the sweet potato and stir to combine.

5. Pour the egg mixture into the skillet and stir to distribute the vegetables evenly.

6. Transfer the skillet to the oven and bake for 15-20 minutes, or until the eggs are set.

7. Remove the skillet from the oven and let it cool for a few minutes.

8. Slice the frittata into wedges and serve with the sweet potato hash on the side.

9. Enjoy!

Nutritional Information:

This meal contains approximately 400 calories, 20 grams of protein, and 15 grams of healthy fats.

Grilled Salmon with Poached Eggs and Avocado

This meal is a delicious and healthy breakfast option that is rich in protein and healthy fats. The salmon provides a great source of protein and omega-3 fatty acids, while the poached eggs and avocado add healthy fats and essential vitamins.

Ingredients:

- 4 oz. salmon fillet
- 2 eggs
- 1 avocado, sliced
- Salt and pepper to taste
- 1 tablespoon olive oil

- 1 tablespoon white vinegar
- 2 cups water

Instructions:

1. Preheat your grill to medium-high heat.

2. Season the salmon fillet with salt and pepper and brush it with olive oil.

3. Grill the salmon for 5-6 minutes per side, or until it is cooked through.

4. While the salmon is cooking, bring a large pot of water to a simmer and add the white vinegar.

5. Crack the eggs into separate bowls and gently pour them into the simmering water. Poach the eggs for 3-4 minutes, or until the whites are set and the yolks are still runny.

6. Remove the poached eggs from the water with a slotted spoon and place them on a paper towel to drain any excess water.

7. Divide the sliced avocado between two plates.

8. Place the grilled salmon on top of the avocado and top each fillet with a poached egg.

9. Season with salt and pepper to taste.

10. Enjoy!

Nutritional Information:

This meal contains approximately 500 calories, 35 grams of protein, and 30 grams of healthy fats.

Recipes For Smoothies And Juices

Strawberry Banana Smoothie with Almond Milk and Chia Seeds

This Strawberry Banana Smoothie is a healthy and delicious drink that is perfect for breakfast or as a refreshing snack. The almond milk adds a creamy texture, while the chia seeds provide an extra boost of protein and omega-3s.

Ingredients:

- 1 cup almond milk
- 1 banana, sliced
- 1 cup strawberries, hulled and halved
- 1 tablespoon chia seeds
- 1 teaspoon honey (optional)

Instructions:

1. Combine almond milk, banana, strawberries, chia seeds, and honey (if using) in a blender.
2. Blend on high speed until smooth and creamy.
3. Pour into a glass and enjoy immediately.

Nutritional Information:

- Calories: 220
- Fat: 6g
- Carbohydrates: 38g
- Fiber: 10g
- Protein: 5g

Green Smoothie with Kale, Pineapple, and Coconut Water

This Green Smoothie is packed with vitamins and nutrients from kale, pineapple, and coconut water. It's a refreshing and energizing drink that will help you start your day on the right foot.

Ingredients:

- 1 cup kale, chopped
- 1 cup frozen pineapple chunks
- 1 cup coconut water
- 1/2 banana (optional)

Instructions:

1. Combine kale, frozen pineapple chunks, coconut water, and banana (if using) in a blender.

2. Blend on high speed until smooth and creamy.

3. Pour into a glass and enjoy immediately.

Nutritional Information:

- Calories: 160
- Fat: 1g
- Carbohydrates: 38g
- Fiber: 6g
- Protein: 4g

Blueberry Lemon Juice with Ginger and Turmeric

This Blueberry Lemon Juice is a refreshing and healthy drink that is packed with antioxidants from blueberries and anti-inflammatory properties from ginger and turmeric. The lemon adds a bright, tangy flavor that balances out the sweetness of the blueberries.

Ingredients:

- 1 cup blueberries

- 1/2 lemon, juiced
- 1/2 inch ginger, peeled and grated
- 1/2 teaspoon turmeric powder
- 1 cup water
- 1 teaspoon honey (optional)

Instructions:

1. Combine blueberries, lemon juice, ginger, turmeric powder, water, and honey (if using) in a blender.

2. Blend on high speed until smooth and well combined.

3. Pour into a glass and enjoy immediately.

Nutritional Information:

- Calories: 80
- Fat: 1g
- Carbohydrates: 21g
- Fiber: 4g
- Protein: 1g

Carrot Apple Juice with Ginger and Cinnamon

This Carrot Apple Juice is a sweet and spicy drink that is perfect for boosting your immune system and providing a burst of energy. The ginger and cinnamon add a warm and spicy flavor to the sweet carrots and apples.

Ingredients:

- 4 carrots, peeled and chopped
- 2 apples, cored and chopped
- 1/2 inch ginger, peeled and grated

- 1/2 teaspoon cinnamon
- 1 cup water
- 1 teaspoon honey (optional)

Instructions:

1. Combine carrots, apples, ginger, cinnamon, water, and honey (if using) in a blender.
2. Blend on high speed until smooth and well combined.
3. Pour into a glass and enjoy immediately.

Nutritional Information:

- Calories: 120
- Fat: 1g
- Carbohydrates: 30g
- Fiber: 6g
- Protein: 1g

Pineapple Ginger Turmeric Shot

This Pineapple Ginger Turmeric Shot is a potent and spicy drink that is perfect for boosting your immune system and fighting inflammation. The combination of pineapple, ginger, and turmeric provides a powerful anti-inflammatory effect that can help reduce pain and swelling in the body.

Ingredients:

- 1 cup pineapple, chopped
- 1/2 inch ginger, peeled and grated
- 1/2 teaspoon turmeric powder

- 1/2 teaspoon black pepper
- 1/4 cup water

Instructions:

1. Combine pineapple, ginger, turmeric powder, black pepper, and water in a blender.

2. Blend on high speed until smooth and well combined.

3. Pour the mixture through a fine mesh strainer to remove any chunks.

4. Drink the liquid immediately in shot glasses.

Nutritional Information:

- Calories: 50
- Fat: 0g
- Carbohydrates: 13g
- Fiber: 2g
- Protein: 1g

Recipes For Low-Carb Breakfast Options

Scrambled eggs with spinach and feta cheese

Description of the meal: Scrambled eggs with spinach and feta cheese is a healthy and delicious breakfast that is easy to make. The combination of fluffy scrambled eggs, sautéed spinach, and tangy feta cheese creates a flavor-packed dish that is sure to satisfy your taste buds.

Ingredients:

- 2 large eggs

- 1/4 cup of fresh spinach leaves
- 1/4 cup of crumbled feta cheese
- 1 tablespoon of olive oil
- Salt and pepper to taste

Instructions:

1. Crack the eggs into a bowl and whisk them together until the yolks and whites are fully combined.

2. Heat the olive oil in a non-stick skillet over medium heat.

3. Add the fresh spinach leaves to the skillet and sauté until they are wilted and tender.

4. Pour the whisked eggs into the skillet with the spinach.

5. Use a spatula to continuously scramble the eggs until they are cooked through and no longer runny.

6. Add the crumbled feta cheese to the skillet and continue to stir until the cheese is melted and evenly distributed throughout the eggs.

7. Season with salt and pepper to taste.

8. Serve hot and enjoy!

Nutritional Information: This recipe makes one serving and contains approximately:

- 250 calories
- 18g of protein
- 19g of fat

- 2g of carbohydrates

Low-carb breakfast burrito with avocado and turkey bacon

Description of the meal: This low-carb breakfast burrito is a delicious and healthy way to start your day. It is packed with protein and healthy fats, and the combination of avocado and turkey bacon creates a creamy and savory flavor.

Ingredients:

- 1 low-carb tortilla
- 2 slices of turkey bacon
- 1/2 of a ripe avocado
- 2 large eggs
- Salt and pepper to taste

Instructions:

1. Cook the turkey bacon in a non-stick skillet over medium heat until crispy.

2. Remove the bacon from the skillet and set it aside.

3. Crack the eggs into the same skillet and cook them until they are scrambled and no longer runny.

4. Warm the low-carb tortilla in the microwave for 15 seconds.

5. Slice the avocado in half and remove the pit.

6. Scoop out the avocado flesh and mash it with a fork.

7. Spread the mashed avocado onto the warmed tortilla.

8. Add the scrambled eggs and turkey bacon to the tortilla.

9. Season with salt and pepper to taste.

10. Roll the tortilla into a burrito shape.

11. Serve hot and enjoy!

Nutritional Information: This recipe makes one serving and contains approximately:

- 350 calories
- 22g of protein
- 23g of fat
- 14g of carbohydrates

Zucchini and egg muffins with cherry tomatoes

Description of the meal: Zucchini and egg muffins with cherry tomatoes are a healthy and flavorful breakfast option that is perfect for on-the-go mornings. These muffins are packed with protein and vegetables, and the cherry tomatoes add a burst of sweetness to each bite.

Ingredients:

- 4 large eggs
- 1 small zucchini, grated
- 1/4 cup of cherry tomatoes, halved
- 1/4 cup of shredded cheddar cheese
- Salt and pepper to taste

Instructions:

1. Preheat the oven to 350°F (175°C).
2. In a large mixing bowl, whisk the eggs together

until the yolks and whites are fully combined.

3. Add the grated zucchini, halved cherry tomatoes, and shredded cheddar cheese to the bowl with the eggs.
4. Mix everything together until well combined.
5. Grease a muffin tin with cooking spray or line with muffin cups.
6. Pour the egg mixture into the muffin cups, filling each one about 2/3 of the way.
7. Bake in the preheated oven for 20-25 minutes or until the muffins are firm to the touch and the tops are lightly golden.
8. Remove the muffins from the oven and allow them to cool for a few minutes.
9. Use a butter knife to loosen the muffins from the edges of the tin or cups, and then remove them from the tin.
10. Serve warm or at room temperature and enjoy!

Nutritional Information: This recipe makes four muffins and each muffin contains approximately:

- 100 calories
- 8g of protein
- 7g of fat
- 2g of carbohydrates

Cottage cheese with chopped nuts and fruit

Description of the meal: Cottage cheese with chopped nuts and fruit is a quick and easy breakfast that is both healthy and delicious. This dish is packed with protein and fiber, and the combination of sweet fruit and crunchy nuts creates a satisfying texture and flavor.

Ingredients:

- 1/2 cup of cottage cheese
- 1/4 cup of chopped nuts (such as almonds, walnuts, or pecans)
- 1/2 cup of fresh fruit (such as berries, sliced banana, or chopped apple)

Instructions:

1. Spoon the cottage cheese into a bowl.
2. Add the chopped nuts and fresh fruit to the bowl.
3. Mix everything together until well combined.
4. Serve and enjoy!

Nutritional Information: This recipe makes one serving and contains approximately:

- 250 calories
- 18g of protein
- 14g of fat
- 14g of carbohydrates

Broccoli and cheese omelette

Description of the meal: Broccoli and cheese omelette is a healthy and flavorful breakfast that is easy to make. The combination of fluffy eggs, tender broccoli, and melted cheese creates a satisfying and delicious meal that is perfect for any morning.

Ingredients:

- 2 large eggs
- 1/2 cup of fresh broccoli florets, chopped

- 1/4 cup of shredded cheddar cheese
- 1 tablespoon of olive oil
- Salt and pepper to taste

Instructions:

1. Crack the eggs into a bowl and whisk them together until the yolks and whites are fully combined.

2. Heat the olive oil in a non-stick skillet over medium heat.

3. Add the chopped broccoli florets to the skillet and sauté until they are tender and slightly browned.

4. Pour the whisked eggs into the skillet with the broccoli.

5. Use a spatula to continuously move the eggs around the skillet, creating a scrambled texture.

6. Once the eggs are nearly cooked, sprinkle the shredded cheddar cheese over the top of the eggs.

7. Use the spatula to fold the omelette in half and allow the cheese to melt inside.

8. Season with salt and pepper to taste.

9. Serve hot and enjoy!

Nutritional Information: This recipe makes one serving and contains approximately:

- 250 calories
- 17g of protein
- 20g of fat
- 3g of carbohydrates

Recipes For High-Fiber Breakfast Options

Overnight Oats with Chia Seeds, Almond Milk, and Banana

This overnight oats recipe is a perfect breakfast for those who have busy mornings but still want to eat healthy. The combination of chia seeds, almond milk, and banana makes for a delicious and satisfying meal.

Ingredients:

- 1/2 cup rolled oats
- 1 tbsp chia seeds
- 1/2 cup almond milk
- 1/2 mashed banana
- 1 tsp honey (optional)

Instructions:

1. Combine rolled oats, chia seeds, and almond milk in a bowl and mix well.

2. Add mashed banana and honey (if desired) to the mixture and stir until fully combined.

3. Cover the bowl with plastic wrap and refrigerate overnight.

4. In the morning, stir the mixture and add toppings such as sliced banana, chopped nuts, and berries.

Nutritional Information:

Calories: 319 | Fat: 9g | Carbohydrates: 53g | Fiber: 12g | Protein: 9g

Bran Muffins with Dried Fruit and Nuts

These bran muffins are packed with fiber and flavor, thanks to the addition of dried fruit and nuts. They make a great on-the-go breakfast or snack.

Ingredients:

- 1 cup wheat bran
- 1 cup all-purpose flour
- 1/4 cup brown sugar
- 1 tsp baking powder
- 1/2 tsp baking soda
- 1/4 tsp salt
- 1/2 cup dried fruit (raisins, cranberries, or cherries)
- 1/2 cup chopped nuts (walnuts, pecans, or almonds)
- 1/2 cup unsweetened applesauce
- 1/2 cup milk
- 1/4 cup vegetable oil
- 1 egg

Instructions:

1. Preheat oven to 375°F and line a muffin tin with paper liners.

2. In a large bowl, mix together wheat bran, all-purpose flour, brown sugar, baking powder, baking soda, and salt.

3. Stir in dried fruit and nuts.

4. In a separate bowl, whisk together applesauce, milk, vegetable oil, and egg.

5. Pour wet ingredients into dry ingredients and mix until just combined.

6. Spoon batter into prepared muffin tin, filling each muffin cup about 2/3 full.

7. Bake for 15-20 minutes, or until a toothpick inserted in the center of a muffin comes out clean.

Nutritional Information:

Calories: 204 | Fat: 8g | Carbohydrates: 31g | Fiber: 5g | Protein: 5g

Avocado Toast with Whole Grain Bread and Mixed Seeds

This avocado toast recipe is a delicious and nutritious breakfast or snack. The combination of creamy avocado and crunchy mixed seeds on whole grain bread is a winner.

Ingredients:

- 2 slices whole grain bread
- 1 avocado
- 1 tbsp lemon juice
- Salt and pepper, to taste
- 1 tbsp mixed seeds (chia, sunflower, pumpkin)

Instructions:

1. Toast the slices of whole grain bread.

2. Cut the avocado in half and remove the pit.

3. Scoop the avocado flesh into a small bowl and add lemon juice, salt, and pepper. Mash the avocado with a fork until smooth.

4. Spread the mashed avocado onto the toasted

bread slices.

5. Sprinkle mixed seeds over the top of the avocado.

Nutritional Information:

Calories: 380 | Fat: 23g | Carbohydrates: 37g | Fiber: 15g | Protein: 11g

Apple Cinnamon Oatmeal with Chopped Walnuts

This apple cinnamon oatmeal recipe is a warm and comforting breakfast option. The addition of chopped walnuts adds a crunchy texture and healthy fats to the meal.

Ingredients:

- 1 cup rolled oats
- 2 cups water
- 1 apple, chopped
- 1 tsp cinnamon
- 1/4 tsp salt
- 1/4 cup chopped walnuts
- 1 tbsp maple syrup (optional)

Instructions:

1. In a medium saucepan, bring water to a boil.

2. Add rolled oats, chopped apple, cinnamon, and salt to the boiling water.

3. Reduce heat to low and simmer for 5-7 minutes, stirring occasionally, until the oats are cooked and the apple is soft.

4. Stir in chopped walnuts and maple syrup (if using).

5. Divide oatmeal into bowls and serve hot.

Nutritional Information:

Calories: 340 | Fat: 11g | Carbohydrates: 55g | Fiber: 9g | Protein: 10g

Smoothie Bowl with Mixed Berries, Spinach, and Almond Butter

This smoothie bowl recipe is a great way to start your day with a healthy and delicious meal. The combination of mixed berries, spinach, and almond butter provides a balanced mix of nutrients and flavors.

Ingredients:

- 1 banana, sliced and frozen
- 1/2 cup mixed berries (strawberries, blueberries, raspberries)
- 1 cup fresh spinach
- 1 tbsp almond butter
- 1/2 cup almond milk
- 1 tbsp honey (optional)
- Toppings: sliced banana, chopped nuts, coconut flakes

Instructions:

1. In a blender, combine frozen banana slices, mixed berries, spinach, almond butter, almond milk, and honey (if using). Blend until smooth.

2. Pour the smoothie mixture into a bowl.

3. Top with sliced banana, chopped nuts, and coconut flakes.

Nutritional Information:

Calories: 356 | Fat: 13g | Carbohydrates: 55g | Fiber: 10g | Protein: 9g

CHAPTER FOUR

Recipes for Lunch and Dinner

Introduction to lunch and dinner recipes for fatty liver disease

Grilled Salmon with Steamed Asparagus and Brown Rice

Description: This meal is a healthy and delicious combination of grilled salmon, steamed asparagus, and brown rice. It is a great source of protein, fiber, and healthy fats.

Ingredients:

- 4 salmon fillets
- 1 bunch of asparagus
- 2 cups of brown rice
- 2 tablespoons of olive oil
- Salt and pepper

Instructions:

1. Cook the brown rice according to the package instructions.
2. Preheat the grill to medium-high heat.
3. Brush the salmon fillets with olive oil and season with salt and pepper.

4. Grill the salmon for 4-5 minutes on each side or until cooked through.

5. While the salmon is grilling, steam the asparagus for 3-4 minutes or until tender.

6. Serve the grilled salmon with steamed asparagus and brown rice.

Nutritional Information:

- Calories: 450
- Protein: 40g
- Fat: 22g
- Carbohydrates: 27g
- Fiber: 5g

Baked Chicken Breast with Roasted Sweet Potatoes and Green Beans

Description: This meal is a healthy and tasty combination of baked chicken breast, roasted sweet potatoes, and green beans. It is a great source of protein, fiber, and vitamins.

Ingredients:

- 4 boneless, skinless chicken breasts
- 2 large sweet potatoes, peeled and diced
- 1 pound of green beans, trimmed
- 2 tablespoons of olive oil
- 2 teaspoons of paprika
- Salt and pepper

Instructions:

1. Preheat the oven to 400°F.

2. Season the chicken breasts with salt, pepper, and paprika.

3. Place the chicken breasts on a baking sheet and bake for 20-25 minutes or until cooked through.

4. While the chicken is baking, toss the sweet potatoes and green beans with olive oil, salt, and pepper.

5. Place the sweet potatoes and green beans on a separate baking sheet and roast for 20-25 minutes or until tender and crispy.

6. Serve the baked chicken breast with roasted sweet potatoes and green beans.

Nutritional Information:

- Calories: 400
- Protein: 40g
- Fat: 12g
- Carbohydrates: 35g
- Fiber: 8g

Turkey Chili with Diced Tomatoes and Mixed Vegetables

Description: This meal is a hearty and flavorful turkey chili made with diced tomatoes and mixed vegetables. It is a great source of protein, fiber, and vitamins.

Ingredients:

- 1 pound of ground turkey
- 1 can of diced tomatoes
- 1 onion, diced

- 2 cloves of garlic, minced
- 1 green bell pepper, diced
- 1 red bell pepper, diced
- 1 zucchini, diced
- 1 teaspoon of cumin
- 1 teaspoon of chili powder
- Salt and pepper

Instructions:

1. Heat a large pot over medium heat.

2. Add the ground turkey and cook until browned.

3. Add the diced tomatoes, onion, garlic, green bell pepper, red bell pepper, zucchini, cumin, chili powder, salt, and pepper.

4. Stir to combine and bring to a boil.

5. Reduce the heat to low and simmer for 20-30 minutes.

6. Serve the turkey chili hot.

Nutritional Information:

- Calories: 350
- Protein: 30g
- Fat: 8g
- Carbohydrates: 25g
- Fiber: 7g

Vegetable Stir-fry with Tofu and Brown Rice

Description: This meal is a healthy and flavorful combination of tofu and mixed vegetables stir-fried with brown rice. It is a great source of protein, fiber, and vitamins.

Ingredients:

- 1 block of tofu, drained and cubed
- 2 cups of mixed vegetables (broccoli, bell pepper, onion, carrot, mushroom)
- 2 cups of cooked brown rice
- 2 tablespoons of soy sauce
- 1 tablespoon of honey
- 1 teaspoon of sesame oil
- Salt and pepper

Instructions:

1. Heat a large skillet or wok over high heat.
2. Add the tofu and stir-fry for 2-3 minutes or until golden brown.
3. Add the mixed vegetables and stir-fry for 2-3 minutes or until tender.
4. In a small bowl, whisk together the soy sauce, honey, sesame oil, salt, and pepper.
5. Add the sauce to the skillet and stir to coat the tofu and vegetables.
6. Serve the vegetable stir-fry hot over cooked brown rice.

Nutritional Information:

- Calories: 400
- Protein: 18g
- Fat: 10g

- Carbohydrates: 60g
- Fiber: 8g

Beef and Broccoli Stir-fry with Quinoa

Description: This meal is a healthy and delicious combination of beef and broccoli stir-fried with quinoa. It is a great source of protein, fiber, and vitamins.

Ingredients:

- 1 pound of flank steak, thinly sliced
- 2 cups of broccoli florets
- 2 cups of cooked quinoa
- 2 tablespoons of soy sauce
- 1 tablespoon of cornstarch
- 1 tablespoon of honey
- 1 teaspoon of sesame oil
- Salt and pepper

Instructions:

1. Heat a large skillet or wok over high heat.
2. Add the sliced beef and stir-fry for 2-3 minutes or until browned.
3. Add the broccoli florets and stir-fry for 2-3 minutes or until tender.
4. In a small bowl, whisk together the soy sauce, cornstarch, honey, sesame oil, salt, and pepper.
5. Add the sauce to the skillet and stir to coat the beef and broccoli.
6. Serve the beef and broccoli stir-fry hot over cooked quinoa.

Nutritional Information:

- Calories: 450
- Protein: 35g
- Fat: 12g
- Carbohydrates: 50g
- Fiber: 8g

Recipes For Lean Protein Options

Grilled Chicken Breast with Roasted Brussels Sprouts and Sweet Potato Mash

Description of the Meal: This is a delicious and healthy meal that is perfect for a satisfying dinner. Grilled chicken breast is seasoned with herbs and served with roasted Brussels sprouts and sweet potato mash.

Ingredients:

- 4 boneless, skinless chicken breasts
- 1 tbsp olive oil
- 1 tsp dried thyme
- 1 tsp dried rosemary
- Salt and pepper
- 1 lb Brussels sprouts, trimmed and halved
- 2 large sweet potatoes, peeled and cubed
- 1/4 cup milk
- 2 tbsp butter

Instructions:

1. Preheat oven to 400°F.

2. In a small bowl, mix olive oil, thyme, rosemary, salt and pepper.

3. Rub the chicken breasts with the herb mixture.

4. Place chicken on a hot grill and cook for 6-7 minutes per side or until cooked through.

5. While the chicken is grilling, toss the Brussels sprouts with olive oil, salt and pepper, and roast in the oven for 20-25 minutes or until tender and golden.

6. Meanwhile, boil the sweet potato cubes until tender, then mash with milk and butter.

7. Serve the grilled chicken with roasted Brussels sprouts and sweet potato mash.

Nutritional Information:

- Calories: 395
- Fat: 12g
- Carbohydrates: 30g
- Protein: 43g
- Fiber: 8g

Baked Salmon with Lemon and Herbs and Sautéed Spinach

Description of the Meal: This baked salmon recipe is packed with flavor from lemon and herbs and served with sautéed spinach for a healthy and nutritious meal.

Ingredients:

- 4 salmon fillets
- 1 lemon, thinly sliced

- 2 tbsp olive oil
- 1 tsp dried thyme
- 1 tsp dried rosemary
- Salt and pepper
- 2 cloves garlic, minced
- 1 lb spinach

Instructions:

1. Preheat oven to 375°F.
2. In a small bowl, mix olive oil, thyme, rosemary, salt and pepper.
3. Rub the salmon fillets with the herb mixture.
4. Place the lemon slices on top of the salmon fillets.
5. Bake for 12-15 minutes or until the salmon is cooked through.
6. While the salmon is baking, heat olive oil in a large skillet over medium heat.
7. Add garlic and cook for 1-2 minutes until fragrant.
8. Add the spinach and cook until wilted, stirring occasionally.
9. Serve the baked salmon with sautéed spinach.

Nutritional Information:

- Calories: 358
- Fat: 23g
- Carbohydrates: 6g
- Protein: 32g

- Fiber: 3g

Turkey and Vegetable Stir-Fry with Brown Rice

Description of the Meal: This quick and easy turkey and vegetable stir-fry is a healthy and delicious meal that is perfect for busy weeknights. Served with brown rice, it is both filling and nutritious.

Ingredients:

- 1 lb ground turkey
- 1 tbsp olive oil
- 1 onion, sliced
- 2 cloves garlic, minced
- 1 red bell pepper, sliced
- 1 yellow bell pepper, sliced
- 2 cups broccoli florets
- 1 cup sliced mushrooms
- 2 tbsp low-sodium soy sauce
- 2 tbsp hoisin sauce
- Salt and pepper
- 3 cups cooked brown rice

Instructions:

1. Heat olive oil in a large skillet or wok over medium-high heat.

2. Add ground turkey and cook until browned, breaking up any large pieces.

3. Add onion, garlic, bell peppers, broccoli, and mushrooms and stir-fry for 5-7 minutes or until vegetables are tender.

4. Add soy sauce and hoisin sauce and stir until everything is evenly coated.

5. Season with salt and pepper to taste.

6. Serve the stir-fry over brown rice.

Nutritional Information:

- Calories: 408
- Fat: 12g
- Carbohydrates: 45g
- Protein: 32g
- Fiber: 7g

Tofu and Vegetable Curry with Quinoa

Description of the Meal: This flavorful tofu and vegetable curry is a healthy and satisfying vegetarian meal. Served with quinoa, it is high in protein and fiber.

Ingredients:

- 1 block firm tofu, cubed
- 1 tbsp olive oil
- 1 onion, diced
- 2 cloves garlic, minced
- 1 red bell pepper, diced
- 1 yellow bell pepper, diced
- 2 cups cauliflower florets
- 1 cup sliced carrots
- 1 can (14 oz) diced tomatoes
- 1 can (14 oz) chickpeas, drained and rinsed
- 1 cup vegetable broth

- 2 tbsp curry powder
- 1 tsp cumin
- Salt and pepper
- 2 cups cooked quinoa

Instructions:

1. Heat olive oil in a large pot or Dutch oven over medium-high heat.

2. Add tofu and cook until browned on all sides, then remove from pot and set aside.

3. Add onion and garlic to the pot and sauté until fragrant, about 1-2 minutes.

4. Add bell peppers, cauliflower, and carrots and sauté for 5-7 minutes or until vegetables are tender.

5. Add diced tomatoes, chickpeas, vegetable broth, curry powder, cumin, salt and pepper and stir to combine.

6. Bring to a boil, then reduce heat and simmer for 15-20 minutes.

7. Serve the curry over quinoa.

Nutritional Information:

- Calories: 393
- Fat: 13g
- Carbohydrates: 50g
- Protein: 23g
- Fiber: 13g

Grilled Shrimp Skewers with Mixed Vegetables and

Quinoa Salad

Description of the Meal: These grilled shrimp skewers are a healthy and flavorful option for a summer barbecue. Served with mixed vegetables and quinoa salad, this meal is both delicious and nutritious.

Ingredients:

- 1 lb large shrimp, peeled and deveined
- 2 tbsp olive oil
- 2 cloves garlic, minced
- 1 tbsp lemon juice
- Salt and pepper
- 1 zucchini, sliced
- 1 yellow squash, sliced
- 1 red onion, sliced
- 2 cups cooked quinoa
- 1 cup cherry tomatoes, halved
- 1/4 cup chopped fresh parsley
- 2 tbsp lemon juice
- 2 tbsp olive oil
- Salt and pepper

Instructions:

1. Preheat grill to medium-high heat.
2. In a small bowl, mix together olive oil, garlic, lemon juice, salt and pepper.
3. Thread shrimp onto skewers, then brush with the garlic and lemon mixture.

4. Grill shrimp skewers for 2-3 minutes per side

5. In a large bowl, mix together zucchini, yellow squash, and red onion. Drizzle with olive oil and season with salt and pepper.

6. Grill the vegetables in a grill basket or wrap in foil and place on the grill for 10-12 minutes, stirring occasionally.

7. In a separate bowl, mix together quinoa, cherry tomatoes, parsley, lemon juice, olive oil, salt and pepper.

8. Serve the grilled shrimp skewers and mixed vegetables over the quinoa salad.

Nutritional Information:

- Calories: 405
- Fat: 16g
- Carbohydrates: 39g
- Protein: 28g
- Fiber: 7g

Recipes For Low-Carb And High-Fiber Options

Grilled Chicken Salad

Description of the Meal: This grilled chicken salad is a light and refreshing meal perfect for a healthy lunch or dinner. It's packed with protein from the chicken and nutritious vegetables, making it a well-balanced meal.

Ingredients:

- 2 boneless, skinless chicken breasts
- 4 cups mixed greens
- 1 cucumber, sliced
- 1 pint cherry tomatoes, halved
- 1/4 cup olive oil
- 2 tablespoons red wine vinegar
- 1 teaspoon Dijon mustard
- Salt and pepper to taste

Instructions:

1. Preheat the grill to medium-high heat.

2. Season the chicken breasts with salt and pepper.

3. Grill the chicken for 6-8 minutes on each side, or until cooked through.

4. Let the chicken rest for 5 minutes before slicing.

5. In a large bowl, combine the mixed greens, cucumber, and cherry tomatoes.

6. In a small bowl, whisk together the olive oil, red wine vinegar, and Dijon mustard to make the dressing.

7. Drizzle the dressing over the salad and toss to combine.

8. Top the salad with the sliced grilled chicken.

Nutritional Information: This grilled chicken salad is low in calories and high in protein, making it a great choice for a healthy meal. One serving contains approximately:

- 300 calories
- 25g protein

- 15g fat
- 15g carbohydrates

Zucchini Noodles with Turkey Meatballs

Description of the Meal: This zucchini noodle dish is a healthier alternative to traditional pasta dishes. The turkey meatballs are a great source of protein, while the zucchini noodles are low in calories and carbs.

Ingredients:

- 4 medium zucchinis, spiralized
- 1 pound ground turkey
- 1/2 cup almond flour
- 1 egg
- 2 cloves garlic, minced
- 1 teaspoon dried oregano
- 1 teaspoon dried basil
- 1/2 teaspoon salt
- 1/4 teaspoon black pepper
- 2 cups marinara sauce

Instructions:

1. Preheat the oven to 400°F.

2. In a large bowl, combine the ground turkey, almond flour, egg, garlic, oregano, basil, salt, and black pepper. Mix well.

3. Form the mixture into small meatballs, about 1 inch in diameter.

4. Place the meatballs on a baking sheet lined with parchment paper and bake for 15-20 minutes, or

until cooked through.

5. While the meatballs are cooking, heat the marinara sauce in a saucepan over medium heat.

6. Add the zucchini noodles to the saucepan and stir until the noodles are coated in the sauce.

7. Serve the zucchini noodles and meatballs together.

Nutritional Information: This zucchini noodle dish is a healthy and satisfying meal. One serving contains approximately:

- 400 calories
- 30g protein
- 20g fat
- 20g carbohydrates

Cauliflower Fried Rice

Description of the Meal: This cauliflower fried rice is a delicious and healthy alternative to traditional fried rice. It's loaded with mixed vegetables and shrimp, making it a well-balanced meal.

Ingredients:

- 1 head cauliflower, riced
- 1 pound shrimp, peeled and deveined
- 2 tablespoons coconut oil
- 1 cup frozen mixed vegetables (peas, carrots, corn, green beans)
- 2 cloves garlic, minced

- 1/4 cup soy sauce

Instructions:

1. Heat a large skillet over medium-high heat.

2. Add the coconut oil to the skillet and swirl to coat the bottom.

3. Add the garlic and sauté for 30 seconds, or until fragrant.

4. Add the shrimp to the skillet and cook for 2-3 minutes on each side, or until pink and cooked through.

5. Remove the shrimp from the skillet and set aside.

6. Add the mixed vegetables to the skillet and cook for 2-3 minutes, or until tender.

7. Add the riced cauliflower to the skillet and stir to combine with the vegetables.

8. Pour the soy sauce over the cauliflower and vegetable mixture and stir to combine.

9. Cook for an additional 2-3 minutes, or until the cauliflower is tender.

10. Add the cooked shrimp back to the skillet and stir to combine.

11. Serve hot.

Nutritional Information: This cauliflower fried rice is a low-carb and low-calorie meal that's packed with protein and nutrients. One serving contains approximately:

- 250 calories
- 25g protein

- 10g fat
- 15g carbohydrates

Broiled Salmon with Steamed Broccoli and Quinoa

Description of the Meal: This broiled salmon dish is a nutritious and satisfying meal. It's paired with steamed broccoli and quinoa for a well-balanced plate.

Ingredients:

- 4 salmon fillets
- 1 tablespoon olive oil
- 1/2 teaspoon salt
- 1/4 teaspoon black pepper
- 2 heads broccoli, chopped
- 1 cup quinoa
- 2 cups water

Instructions:

1. Preheat the broiler to high.
2. Place the salmon fillets on a baking sheet lined with parchment paper.
3. Drizzle the olive oil over the salmon fillets and season with salt and black pepper.
4. Broil the salmon for 8-10 minutes, or until cooked through.
5. While the salmon is cooking, bring 2 cups of water to a boil in a medium saucepan.
6. Add the quinoa to the saucepan and stir to combine.

7. Reduce the heat to low, cover the saucepan, and simmer for 15-20 minutes, or until the quinoa is tender and the water has been absorbed.

8. Steam the chopped broccoli in a steamer basket for 5-7 minutes, or until tender.

9. Serve the broiled salmon with the steamed broccoli and cooked quinoa.

Nutritional Information: This broiled salmon dish is a great source of protein and healthy fats. Paired with steamed broccoli and quinoa, it's a well-balanced meal. One serving contains approximately:

- 450 calories
- 35g protein
- 20g fat
- 35g carbohydrates

Turkey Chili

Description of the Meal: This turkey chili is a hearty and healthy meal that's perfect for a cold night. Loaded with mixed beans and diced tomatoes, it's packed with nutrients and flavor.

Ingredients:

- 1 pound ground turkey
- 1 tablespoon olive oil
- 1 onion, chopped
- 2 cloves garlic, minced
- 1 tablespoon chili powder
- 1 teaspoon ground cumin
- 1/2 teaspoon salt

- 1/4 teaspoon black pepper
- 1 can (15 ounces) kidney beans, drained and rinsed
- 1 can (15 ounces) black beans, drained and rinsed
- 1 can (15 ounces) diced tomatoes

Instructions:

1. Heat the olive oil in a large pot over medium-high heat.

2. Add the chopped onion and sauté for 2-3 minutes, or until softened.

3. Add the minced garlic and sauté for an additional 30 seconds, or until fragrant.

4. Add the ground turkey to the pot and cook, breaking it up with a spatula, until browned and cooked through.

5. Add the chili powder, ground cumin, salt, and black pepper to the pot and stir to combine.

6. Add the kidney beans, black beans, and diced tomatoes to the pot and stir to combine.

7. Bring the mixture to a simmer and cook for 15-20 minutes, or until the chili is heated through and the flavors have melded together.

8. Serve hot, garnished with your favorite toppings, such as shredded cheese, diced avocado, or chopped cilantro.

Nutritional Information: This turkey chili is a nutritious and satisfying meal that's high in protein and fiber. One serving contains approximately:

- 350 calories
- 30g protein
- 10g fat
- 35g carbohydrates
- 15g fiber

Recipes For Healthy Fats Options

Grilled Salmon with Avocado and Mixed Greens Salad

Description

This meal is a delicious combination of grilled salmon and creamy avocado paired with a refreshing mixed greens salad.

Ingredients

- 2 salmon fillets
- 2 avocados, sliced
- 4 cups mixed greens
- 1/4 cup cherry tomatoes, halved
- 2 tablespoons olive oil
- Salt and pepper, to taste

Instructions

1. Preheat grill to medium-high heat.
2. Brush salmon fillets with olive oil and season with salt and pepper.
3. Grill salmon for 4-5 minutes on each side or until cooked through.
4. In a large mixing bowl, combine mixed greens,

cherry tomatoes, and sliced avocado.

5. Drizzle olive oil over the salad and toss to coat.

6. Serve grilled salmon over the mixed greens salad.

Nutritional Information

This meal is packed with healthy fats and protein. It contains approximately 450 calories per serving.

Baked Chicken Breast with Roasted Brussels Sprouts and Mashed Avocado

Description

This meal features tender baked chicken breast served with roasted Brussels sprouts and creamy mashed avocado.

Ingredients

- 2 chicken breasts
- 1 pound Brussels sprouts, halved
- 2 avocados
- 2 tablespoons olive oil
- Salt and pepper, to taste

Instructions

1. Preheat oven to 375°F.

2. Place chicken breasts in a baking dish and season with salt and pepper.

3. Bake chicken for 25-30 minutes or until cooked through.

4. Toss Brussels sprouts with olive oil, salt, and pepper.

5. Roast Brussels sprouts in the oven for 20-25 minutes or until tender.

6. In a mixing bowl, mash avocados and season with salt and pepper.

7. Serve baked chicken breast with roasted Brussels sprouts and mashed avocado.

Nutritional Information

This meal is high in protein and healthy fats. It contains approximately 500 calories per serving.

Tuna Salad with Mixed Greens, Avocado, and Cherry Tomatoes

Description

This meal is a refreshing and satisfying tuna salad served with mixed greens, creamy avocado, and juicy cherry tomatoes.

Ingredients

- 2 cans of tuna, drained
- 2 avocados, sliced
- 4 cups mixed greens
- 1/4 cup cherry tomatoes, halved
- 2 tablespoons olive oil
- Salt and pepper, to taste

Instructions

1. In a mixing bowl, combine tuna, sliced avocado, and cherry tomatoes.

2. Season with salt and pepper.

3. In a large mixing bowl, combine mixed greens and tuna mixture.

4. Drizzle olive oil over the salad and toss to coat.

5. Serve tuna salad with mixed greens and avocado.

Nutritional Information

This meal is high in protein and healthy fats. It contains approximately 400 calories per serving.

Grilled Shrimp with Mixed Vegetables and Avocado Salsa

Description

This meal is a flavorful combination of grilled shrimp, mixed vegetables, and creamy avocado salsa.

Ingredients

- 1 pound shrimp, peeled and deveined
- 2 avocados, diced
- 1 red bell pepper, sliced
- 1 yellow bell pepper, sliced
- 1 zucchini, sliced
- 1 tablespoon olive oil
- Salt and pepper, to taste

Instructions

1. Preheat grill to medium-high heat.

2. In a mixing bowl, toss shrimp with olive oil, salt, and pepper.

3. Grill shrimp for 2-3 minutes on each side

4. In a separate mixing bowl, combine diced

avocado, sliced red and yellow bell peppers, and sliced zucchini.

5. Season with salt and pepper and toss to combine.

6. Grill mixed vegetables in a grilling basket for 8-10 minutes or until tender.

7. Serve grilled shrimp with mixed vegetables and avocado salsa on top.

Nutritional Information

This meal is low in calories and high in protein. It contains approximately 300 calories per serving.

Baked Salmon with Roasted Asparagus and Mashed Sweet Potatoes with Olive Oil

Description

This meal is a delicious and nutritious combination of baked salmon, roasted asparagus, and mashed sweet potatoes with a drizzle of olive oil.

Ingredients

- 2 salmon fillets
- 1 pound asparagus
- 2 sweet potatoes, peeled and cubed
- 2 tablespoons olive oil
- Salt and pepper, to taste

Instructions

1. Preheat oven to 375°F.

2. Place salmon fillets in a baking dish and season with salt and pepper.

3. Bake salmon for 12-15 minutes or until cooked through.

4. Toss asparagus with olive oil, salt, and pepper.

5. Roast asparagus in the oven for 10-12 minutes or until tender.

6. Boil sweet potatoes in a pot of water for 10-12 minutes or until tender.

7. Drain sweet potatoes and mash with a fork.

8. Drizzle olive oil over mashed sweet potatoes and season with salt and pepper.

9. Serve baked salmon with roasted asparagus and mashed sweet potatoes.

Nutritional Information

This meal is high in protein and fiber. It contains approximately 400 calories per serving.

CHAPTER FIVE

Recipes for Snacks and Desserts

Introduction to snack and dessert recipes for fatty liver disease

Apple slices with almond butter and cinnamon

Description: This delicious snack is a perfect combination of sweet and savory flavors. Crisp apple slices are paired with creamy almond butter and a sprinkle of warm cinnamon, making it a healthy and satisfying snack that's easy to make.

Ingredients:

- 1 medium-sized apple, sliced
- 1 tablespoon almond butter
- 1/4 teaspoon cinnamon

Instructions:

1. Wash the apple and slice it into thin pieces.
2. Spread the almond butter on the slices of apple.
3. Sprinkle cinnamon on top of the almond butter.
4. Enjoy your delicious snack!

Nutritional Information:

- Calories: 140

- Fat: 6g
- Carbohydrates: 22g
- Protein: 2g
- Fiber: 4g

Greek yogurt with fresh berries and a sprinkle of granola

Description: This breakfast or snack idea is not only delicious, but also packed with protein and fiber to keep you feeling full and satisfied. The tangy Greek yogurt pairs perfectly with the sweetness of fresh berries, and the crunchy granola adds a satisfying texture.

Ingredients:

- 1/2 cup Greek yogurt
- 1/2 cup fresh berries (such as blueberries, strawberries, or raspberries)
- 1/4 cup granola

Instructions:

1. In a bowl, spoon the Greek yogurt.
2. Add the fresh berries on top of the yogurt.
3. Sprinkle the granola over the berries.
4. Enjoy your delicious and nutritious breakfast or snack!

Nutritional Information:

- Calories: 220
- Fat: 6g
- Carbohydrates: 31g
- Protein: 14g

- Fiber: 5g

Baked sweet potato fries with a side of hummus

Description: These sweet potato fries are baked, not fried, making them a healthier alternative to traditional French fries. The natural sweetness of the sweet potato pairs well with the creamy and savory hummus for a delicious and satisfying snack or side dish.

Ingredients:

- 1 medium-sized sweet potato
- 1 tablespoon olive oil
- 1/4 teaspoon salt
- 1/4 teaspoon paprika
- 1/4 teaspoon garlic powder
- 1/4 cup hummus

Instructions:

1. Preheat the oven to 425°F (220°C).
2. Peel the sweet potato and cut it into thin strips.
3. In a bowl, toss the sweet potato strips with olive oil, salt, paprika, and garlic powder.
4. Spread the sweet potato strips out in a single layer on a baking sheet.
5. Bake for 20-25 minutes, or until crispy and golden brown.
6. Serve with a side of hummus for dipping.

Nutritional Information:

- Calories: 240
- Fat: 10g
- Carbohydrates: 32g
- Protein: 6g
- Fiber: 7g

Roasted chickpeas with a dash of paprika and garlic powder

Description: These roasted chickpeas are a crunchy and protein-packed snack that's perfect for any time of day. The smoky and savory flavor of paprika and garlic powder adds a delicious twist to this healthy snack.

Ingredients:

- 1 can (15 ounces) chickpeas, drained and rinsed
- 1 tablespoon olive oil
- 1/4 teaspoon salt
- 1/4 teaspoon paprika
- 1/4 teaspoon garlic powder

Instructions:

1. Preheat the oven to 400°F (200°C).
2. In a bowl, toss the chickpeas with olive oil, salt, paprika, and garlic powder.
3. Spread the chickpeas out in a single layer on a baking sheet.
4. Roast for 20-25 minutes, or until crispy and golden brown.
5. Let the chickpeas cool for a few minutes before

serving.

Nutritional Information:

- Calories: 140
- Fat: 6g
- Carbohydrates: 16g
- Protein: 6g
- Fiber: 5g

Carrot sticks with a low-fat yogurt dip

Description: Carrots are not only delicious, but also packed with vitamins and minerals. Paired with a low-fat yogurt dip, this snack is a great way to add more vegetables into your diet.

Ingredients:

- 2-3 medium-sized carrots, peeled and cut into sticks
- 1/4 cup plain low-fat yogurt
- 1/4 teaspoon garlic powder
- 1/4 teaspoon dried dill
- 1/4 teaspoon salt

Instructions:

1. Wash and peel the carrots, then cut them into sticks.

2. In a small bowl, mix together the low-fat yogurt, garlic powder, dried dill, and salt.

3. Serve the carrot sticks with the yogurt dip on the side.

Nutritional Information:

- Calories: 70
- Fat: 1g
- Carbohydrates: 13g
- Protein: 3g
- Fiber: 3g

Recipes for healthy snack options

Air-popped popcorn with a sprinkle of nutritional yeast

Description of the meal

Air-popped popcorn with a sprinkle of nutritional yeast is a healthy and delicious snack that is perfect for movie nights or a quick snack break. This recipe is gluten-free, vegan and packed with vitamins and minerals.

Ingredients

- 1/2 cup of popcorn kernels
- 2 tablespoons of nutritional yeast
- Salt to taste

Instruction

1. Place the popcorn kernels in a paper bag and fold over the top a few times.

2. Microwave on high for 2-3 minutes, or until the popping slows down.

3. Remove the popcorn from the microwave and pour it into a large bowl.

4. Sprinkle the nutritional yeast and salt over the

popcorn and toss well to combine.

5. Serve and enjoy.

Nutritional Information

- Calories: 120
- Protein: 4g
- Fat: 2g
- Carbohydrates: 22g
- Fiber: 4g

Sliced cucumber with a hummus dip

Description of the meal

Sliced cucumber with a hummus dip is a refreshing and healthy snack that is perfect for hot summer days or as an appetizer for a party. This recipe is vegan, gluten-free and packed with vitamins and minerals.

Ingredients

- 1 cucumber, sliced
- 1 cup of hummus

Instruction

1. Wash the cucumber and slice it into rounds.
2. Place the hummus in a bowl and serve it with the cucumber slices.

Nutritional Information

- Calories: 150
- Protein: 7g
- Fat: 10g

- Carbohydrates: 11g
- Fiber: 4g

Hard-boiled eggs with a side of baby carrots

Description of the meal

Hard-boiled eggs with a side of baby carrots is a protein-packed and easy-to-make snack that is perfect for on-the-go or as a quick breakfast. This recipe is gluten-free and low-carb.

Ingredients

- 2 hard-boiled eggs
- 1 cup of baby carrots

Instruction

1. Peel the hard-boiled eggs and slice them in half.
2. Arrange the eggs and baby carrots on a plate.
3. Serve and enjoy.

Nutritional Information

- Calories: 180
- Protein: 12g
- Fat: 12g
- Carbohydrates: 7g
- Fiber: 2g

Cherry tomatoes with a drizzle of balsamic vinegar and olive oil

Description of the meal

Cherry tomatoes with a drizzle of balsamic vinegar and olive oil is a simple and delicious snack that is perfect for a mid-day snack or as a side dish for a meal. This recipe is vegan, gluten-free and packed with vitamins and antioxidants.

Ingredients

- 1 cup of cherry tomatoes
- 1 tablespoon of balsamic vinegar
- 1 tablespoon of olive oil

Instruction

1. Wash the cherry tomatoes and slice them in half.
2. Place the cherry tomatoes in a bowl.
3. Drizzle the balsamic vinegar and olive oil over the tomatoes.
4. Toss well to combine.
5. Serve and enjoy.

Nutritional Information

- Calories: 80
- Protein: 1g
- Fat: 7g
- Carbohydrates: 4g
- Fiber: 1g

Homemade trail mix with mixed nuts, seeds, and dried fruit

Description of the meal

Homemade trail mix with mixed nuts, seeds, and dried

fruit is a healthy and easy-to-make snack that is perfect for hiking, camping or as a mid-day snack.

Ingredients

- 1 cup of mixed nuts (almonds, cashews, walnuts)
- 1/2 cup of mixed seeds (pumpkin seeds, sunflower seeds)
- 1/2 cup of dried fruit (raisins, cranberries, apricots)

Instruction

1. Combine the mixed nuts, mixed seeds and dried fruit in a bowl.
2. Toss well to combine.
3. Store the trail mix in an airtight container.

Nutritional Information

- Calories: 180
- Protein: 6g
- Fat: 12g
- Carbohydrates: 15g
- Fiber: 3g

Note: Nutritional information may vary based on the specific ingredients used in the recipe. It's important to read labels and choose high-quality ingredients to ensure the best nutritional value.

Recipes For Low-Sugar And Low-Fat Dessert Options

Baked Apples with Cinnamon and a Drizzle of Honey

This delicious dessert is perfect for those who want to satisfy their sweet tooth without indulging in a heavy dessert. Baked apples are healthy and packed with flavor.

Ingredients:

- 4 large apples
- 1 tablespoon cinnamon
- 1 tablespoon honey
- 1 tablespoon coconut oil

Instructions:

1. Preheat your oven to 375°F (190°C).
2. Cut off the top of the apples and scoop out the seeds.
3. Place the apples in a baking dish.
4. Mix the cinnamon and coconut oil together and rub the mixture over the apples.
5. Drizzle honey over the top of the apples.
6. Bake in the oven for 30-35 minutes or until the apples are tender.
7. Serve warm with a scoop of vanilla ice cream (optional).

Nutritional Information:

This recipe serves 4 people and each serving contains approximately:

- Calories: 121
- Fat: 3g
- Carbohydrates: 26g

- Protein: 1g
- Fiber: 4g

Greek Yogurt with Mixed Berries and a Sprinkle of Chopped Nuts

This breakfast is packed with protein and antioxidants, making it a great way to start your day. Greek yogurt is thick and creamy, while the mixed berries and chopped nuts add a variety of textures and flavors.

Ingredients:

- 1 cup Greek yogurt
- 1/2 cup mixed berries
- 2 tablespoons chopped nuts

Instructions:

1. In a bowl, mix the Greek yogurt until it is smooth and creamy.
2. Top the Greek yogurt with mixed berries and chopped nuts.
3. Serve immediately.

Nutritional Information:

This recipe serves 1 person and contains approximately:

- Calories: 232
- Fat: 10g
- Carbohydrates: 17g
- Protein: 20g
- Fiber: 3g

Chia Seed Pudding with Almond Milk and Fresh Fruit

This healthy dessert is perfect for those who want to indulge in a sweet treat without any guilt. Chia seeds are packed with fiber and omega-3 fatty acids, while almond milk is low in calories and high in calcium.

Ingredients:

- 1/4 cup chia seeds
- 1 cup unsweetened almond milk
- 1/2 teaspoon vanilla extract
- 1 tablespoon maple syrup
- 1/2 cup fresh fruit

Instructions:

1. In a bowl, mix the chia seeds, almond milk, vanilla extract, and maple syrup.
2. Cover the bowl and refrigerate overnight.
3. In the morning, mix the chia seed pudding again to break up any clumps.
4. Top the chia seed pudding with fresh fruit and serve.

Nutritional Information:

This recipe serves 2 people and each serving contains approximately:

- Calories: 140
- Fat: 7g
- Carbohydrates: 17g

- Protein: 5g
- Fiber: 11g

Banana Oatmeal Cookies with Unsweetened Applesauce

These cookies are a healthy and delicious snack that are perfect for any time of day. They are packed with fiber, potassium, and protein, making them a great option for anyone who wants to satisfy their sweet tooth without indulging in a heavy dessert.

Ingredients:

- 2 ripe bananas, mashed
- 1 cup old-fashioned oats
- 1/2 cup unsweetened applesauce
- 1/4 cup almond butter
- 1/4 cup raisins

Instructions:

1. Pre-heat your oven to 350°F (175°C). 2. In a mixing bowl, combine the mashed bananas, oats, applesauce, almond butter, and raisins.

3. Mix well until all the ingredients are well combined.

4. Using a cookie scoop or spoon, drop the cookie dough onto a baking sheet lined with parchment paper.

5. Flatten the dough with a fork to create a cookie shape.

6. Bake for 12-15 minutes or until golden brown.

7. Remove from the oven and let them cool before serving.

Nutritional Information:

This recipe makes 12 cookies and each cookie contains approximately:

- Calories: 97
- Fat: 3g
- Carbohydrates: 17g
- Protein: 2g
- Fiber: 2g

Chocolate Avocado Mousse with Cocoa Powder and a Touch of Maple Syrup

This healthy dessert is perfect for chocolate lovers who want to indulge in a guilt-free treat. Avocado is the secret ingredient that makes this mousse creamy and smooth, while cocoa powder and maple syrup add a rich and decadent flavor.

Ingredients:

- 2 ripe avocados
- 1/2 cup cocoa powder
- 1/4 cup maple syrup
- 1/4 cup unsweetened almond milk
- 1/2 teaspoon vanilla extract

Instructions:

1. Cut the avocados in half, remove the pit, and scoop out the flesh into a blender.
2. Add the cocoa powder, maple syrup, almond milk,

and vanilla extract to the blender.

3. Blend all the ingredients until they are smooth and creamy.

4. Pour the mousse into individual cups and refrigerate for at least 1 hour before serving.

5. Top with fresh berries or chopped nuts, if desired.

Nutritional Information:

This recipe serves 4 people and each serving contains approximately:

- Calories: 219
- Fat: 15g
- Carbohydrates: 26g
- Protein: 4g
- Fiber: 8g

CONCLUSION

Recap Of The Importance Of A Healthy Diet In Managing Fatty Liver Disease

Fatty liver disease is a condition that occurs when there is an accumulation of excess fat in the liver. This condition can be caused by a variety of factors, including obesity, type 2 diabetes, and high blood pressure. Fatty liver disease can be divided into two categories: alcoholic fatty liver disease (AFLD) and non-alcoholic fatty liver disease (NAFLD). AFLD is caused by excessive alcohol consumption, while NAFLD is caused by factors such as obesity and insulin resistance.

While the causes of fatty liver disease are varied, one of the most effective ways to manage the condition is through diet. A healthy diet is essential for maintaining liver health and preventing further damage to the liver. There are several dietary recommendations that can help manage fatty liver disease:

- **Reduce calorie intake**: One of the primary causes of fatty liver disease is obesity. Therefore, it is essential to reduce calorie intake and achieve a healthy weight. A calorie-restricted diet has been shown to improve liver function in patients with fatty liver disease.

- **Limit sugar intake**: Excess sugar consumption is linked to the development of fatty liver disease.

Therefore, it is essential to limit sugar intake by avoiding sugary drinks and snacks.

- **Increase fiber intake**: A high-fiber diet has been shown to improve liver function in patients with fatty liver disease. Therefore, it is important to increase fiber intake by consuming fruits, vegetables, and whole grains.

- **Avoid alcohol**: Alcohol consumption is a major cause of AFLD. Therefore, it is important to avoid alcohol consumption or limit it to moderate levels.

- **Increase protein intake**: Adequate protein intake is important for liver function. However, it is important to choose lean protein sources such as fish, chicken, and beans.

- **Avoid processed foods**: Processed foods are high in fat, sugar, and calories, which can exacerbate fatty liver disease. Therefore, it is important to avoid processed foods and opt for whole foods instead.

In addition to dietary changes, physical activity is also an important factor in managing fatty liver disease. Regular exercise can help improve liver function, reduce inflammation, and improve insulin sensitivity. Therefore, it is important to engage in regular physical activity, such as walking, cycling, or swimming.

Overall, a healthy diet and lifestyle are essential for managing fatty liver disease. By making dietary changes and engaging in regular physical activity, patients with fatty liver disease can improve liver function and prevent further liver damage.

Final thoughts and encouragement for maintaining a healthy lifestyle

Maintaining a healthy lifestyle is essential for overall health and well-being. In addition to managing fatty liver disease, a healthy lifestyle can help prevent a variety of chronic diseases, including heart disease, diabetes, and cancer. Therefore, it is important to prioritize healthy habits in daily life.

Here are some final thoughts and encouragement for maintaining a healthy lifestyle:

- **Make small changes**: Maintaining a healthy lifestyle doesn't have to be overwhelming. Start by making small changes to your diet and lifestyle, such as adding more fruits and vegetables to your diet or taking a daily walk.

- **Find an activity you enjoy**: Physical activity is an important aspect of a healthy lifestyle. However, it can be challenging to stay motivated if you don't enjoy the activity. Find an activity that you enjoy, such as dancing, hiking, or playing a sport.

- **Get support**: Maintaining a healthy lifestyle can be challenging, especially if you are making significant changes to your diet and lifestyle. Get support from friends, family, or a healthcare professional to help you stay motivated and on track.

- **Stay hydrated**: Drinking enough water is essential for overall health and can help support healthy liver function. Aim for at least 8 cups of water per day.

- **Focus on nutrient-dense foods**: Rather than focusing on calorie counting or restrictive diets, aim to consume nutrient-dense foods such as fruits, vegetables, lean proteins, and whole grains. These foods provide essential vitamins and minerals that support overall health and well-being.

- **Practice mindful eating**: Mindful eating involves being present and fully engaged in the eating experience. This can help you make healthier food choices and prevent overeating.

Remember, maintaining a healthy lifestyle is a journey, not a destination. It's important to be kind to yourself and celebrate small successes along the way. By prioritizing healthy habits and making small changes to your diet and lifestyle, you can improve your overall health and well-being.

Additional resources for managing fatty liver disease

Managing fatty liver disease can be challenging, especially if you are unsure where to turn for support and resources. Fortunately, there are several resources available to help you manage the condition and improve your overall health.

- **Healthcare professionals**: Your healthcare provider can provide guidance and support for managing fatty liver disease. They can help you develop a personalized treatment plan and monitor your progress over time.

- **Registered dietitians**: Registered dietitians are experts in nutrition and can provide guidance on making dietary changes to manage fatty liver disease. They can help you develop a meal plan that meets your individual needs and preferences.

- **Support groups**: Joining a support group can provide emotional support and help you connect with others who are going through similar experiences. Ask your healthcare provider or search online for support groups in your area.

- **Online resources**: There are several online resources available for managing fatty liver disease, including educational materials, recipes, and support forums. Some reputable websites include the American Liver Foundation and the National Institute of Diabetes and Digestive and Kidney Diseases.